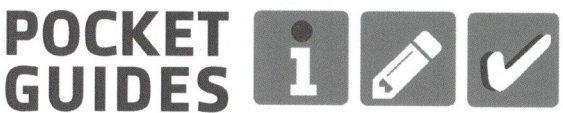

POCKET
GUIDES

W0037662

PHYSIOTHERAPY PLACEMENTS

Pocket Guides

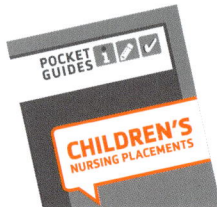

"A very useful, well-written and practical pocket book for any level of student nurse preparing for clinical placement. This book is also a great resource for lecturers and mentors to have, to help students get the most out of their placement time." ★★★★★

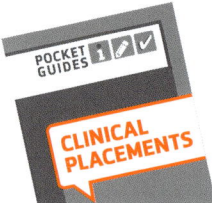

"This is such a useful guide that has just the right amount of need to know info for student nurses on clinical placement, as well as loads of little tips scattered throughout. A must-have for student nurses on placements!"
★★★★★

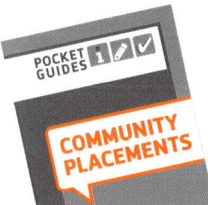

"Full of everything you need to know as a student nurse on placement. Written by students for students. Helpful little references to help with abbreviations and common medications. A must for any student about to head on placement."
★★★★★

Forthcoming:

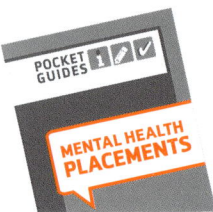

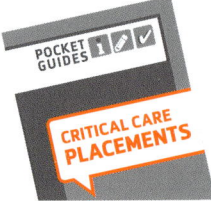

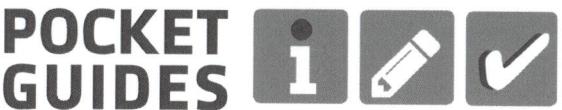

POCKET GUIDES

PHYSIOTHERAPY PLACEMENTS

Fiona Moffatt, Ben Bradley and Laura Loeber

University of Nottingham

Lantern

ISBN: 9781908625694
First published in 2020 by Lantern Publishing Ltd

Lantern Publishing Limited, The Old Hayloft, Vantage
Business Park, Bloxham Road, Banbury OX16 9UX, UK
www.lanternpublishing.com

British Library Cataloguing in Publication Data
A catalogue record for this book is available from the British Library

The authors and publisher have made every attempt to ensure
the content of this book is up to date and accurate. However,
healthcare knowledge and information is changing all the time
so the reader is advised to double-check any information in
this text on drug usage, treatment procedures, the use of
equipment, etc. to confirm that it complies with the latest safety
recommendations, standards of practice and legislation, as well as
local Trust policies and procedures. Students are advised to check
with their tutor and/or practice supervisor before carrying out
any of the procedures in this textbook.

Typeset by Medlar Publishing Solutions Pvt Ltd, India
Printed and bound in the UK

Last digit is the print number: 10 9 8 7 6 5 4

Personal information

Name:..

Mobile number:....................................

University contact details:.........................

Personal tutor details:............................

....

CONTACT IN CASE OF EMERGENCY

Name:..

Mobile number:....................................

Home/work numbers:..............................

....

Contents

Acknowledgements

The authors would like to thank all the individuals who have contributed to the development of this book:

- The wonderful physiotherapy students of the University of Nottingham who have reviewed draft outlines and contributed to focus groups
- Sian Keane, Anna Lord and James Clayton for their direct contributions
- Kirsty Hyndes, Jackie Hollowell, Eleanor Douglas, Dr Leigh Campbell and Dr Roger Kerry
- The University of Nottingham Clinical Placement Team (past and present)
- Joss Moffatt for his IT skills

The publishers would like to thank Kirstie Paterson and Jessica Wallar, authors of *Clinical Placements*, the first in the Pocket Guides series, and Kath MacDonald, their editor, for permission to use some of the content from their book as well as the overall framework.

Abbreviations

Below you will find abbreviations used in this book. There is also space for you to create a list of further (approved) abbreviations that you encounter during placement. Familiarise yourself with locally approved abbreviations in your first few days of placement.

A&E	Accident and Emergency Department (also referred to as Emergency Department [ED] or Emergency Room [ER])
ABCDE	Airway, Breathing, Circulation, Disability, Exposure
ABG	Arterial blood gas
ACVPU	Alert, confused, responds to voice/touch, responds to pain, unresponsive
BE	Base excess
BEG	Beliefs, expectations, goals
BLS	Basic Life Support
BP	Blood pressure
COPD	Chronic obstructive pulmonary disease
CPD	Continuing professional development
CSP	Chartered Society of Physiotherapy
DH	Drug history
DVT	Deep vein thrombosis (You should also be aware of the acronym VTE – venous thromboembolism. This refers to the formation of a blood clot in a vein [DVT] which can dislodge and travel to the pulmonary arteries causing a pulmonary embolus [PE])
FAQ	Frequently asked questions
FEV_1	Forced expiratory volume in 1 second
FVC	Forced vital capacity
HCO_3^-	Bicarbonate ions
HCPC	Health and Care Professions Council

HIV	Human immunodeficiency virus
HPC	History of present condition
HR	Heart rate
MDT	Multidisciplinary team
MND	Motor neurone disease
MRC	Medical Research Council
MS	Multiple sclerosis
MSK OP	Musculoskeletal outpatients
NEWS2	National Early Warning Score
NICE	National Institute for Health and Care Excellence
OA	Osteoarthritis
OT	Occupational therapy
$PaCO_2$	Partial pressure of carbon dioxide in arterial blood
PaO_2	Partial pressure of oxygen in arterial blood
PC	Present condition
PCC	Person-centred care
PEFR	Peak expiratory flow rate
PMH	Past medical history
PPE	Personal protective equipment
RA	Rheumatoid arthritis
ROM	Range of movement
RR	Respiratory rate
SBAR	Situation, background, assessment, recommendation
SH	Social history
SpO_2	Oxygen saturations
SWOT	Strengths, weaknesses, opportunities, threats
TILE	Task, individual, load, environment

Note your own (approved) abbreviations

Notes

Before you go

Preparing for placement

ℹ️ Top tip

First placements can be daunting. Being as prepared as possible can help you cope with many of your worries and anxieties. This guide is designed to help you prepare so you can then get the most out of your placements.

With all the new stressors and change in routine it can be easy to forget to look after yourself. It is worth thinking about how you will manage in advance:

- Get plenty of rest
- Eat healthy, easily prepared meals; stock up on shopping
- Plan some relaxation time; go to the gym or meet a friend.

✔️ Checklist six weeks before placement

- ☐ *Get the details of your placement provider from your university placement team*
- ☐ *Contact your placement provider to confirm the placement and obtain your educator details*
- ☐ *Email your educator with your personal details and check:*
  - ☐ *what type of unit it is*
  - ☐ *where it is located in the hospital/health centre*
  - ☐ *working hours/shift patterns*
  - ☐ *where to meet on the first day and at what time*
  - ☐ *if you require an NHS Smartcard*
  - ☐ *uniform requirements*

- [ ] changing facilities
- [ ] lunch arrangements
- [ ] Follow your placement provider's policy for obtaining an NHS Smartcard (if required). You will need to provide the following:
  - [ ] your date of birth
  - [ ] your National Insurance Number
  - [ ] photographic ID (×2)
  - [ ] proof of address (×2)
- [ ] Are any other students on placement at the same organisation? If so, liaise with them and see if it is practicable for you to travel together
- [ ] Arrange your travel plans; if possible, do a practice run by bus, car or train remembering that weekend timetables and rush hour travel will be different. Have a back-up plan if you are relying on a lift. Find out about parking arrangements, and if you are using your own car check that you have appropriate insurance
- [ ] Book accommodation if you need to live away. Your university placement team may be able to assist with this
- [ ] Revise – find out as much as possible about the type of work you will be doing before you start. Your educator will guide you. It may be helpful to have some information about typical patient groups/patient flow for that department or unit
- [ ] Disclose – if you have any additional learning needs or personal issues that you feel may impact on placement it is good practice to inform your educator as soon as possible. This will give them the opportunity to make any reasonable adjustments that may help you. If you are unsure about this speak to your university placement team or personal tutor.

✔ Checklist of things to bring on your first day

- ☐ *Your uniform and shoes*
- ☐ *Hair ties if appropriate*
- ☐ *Pocket notebook and black pens*
- ☐ *Water bottle*
- ☐ *Food or money to buy lunch*
- ☐ *This handbook*

Notes

As a student you will have been supplied with the appropriate uniform to wear by your university. Wear your uniform with pride and remember it represents your profession. Your uniform may be formal tunic and trousers, or more practical wear such as a polo shirt, depending on the location of your placement.

Your responsibilities to meet infection control compliance and safety standards include:

- Always wear your name badge
- Hair should be tied back and off the collar; beards/moustaches neatly trimmed
- Nails short and clean (no artificial, painted or gel nails)
- Minimal, natural make-up
- Uniform should not be worn travelling to and from placement
- No jewellery or watches should be worn other than a plain ring (some placements may permit you to wear a religious bangle)
- No undershirts to be below the elbow
- All uniform to be clean and ironed, and laundered appropriately
- Shoes must be clean and smart and not put the wearer at risk of injury (most uniform policy specifies dark shoes with a contained toe; some placements may allow trainers if appropriate)
- Tattoos which may cause offence need to be covered
- Please check local uniform policy regarding piercings

These policies are in place to protect our patients, ourselves and other healthcare professionals.

Students are expected to look professional at all times

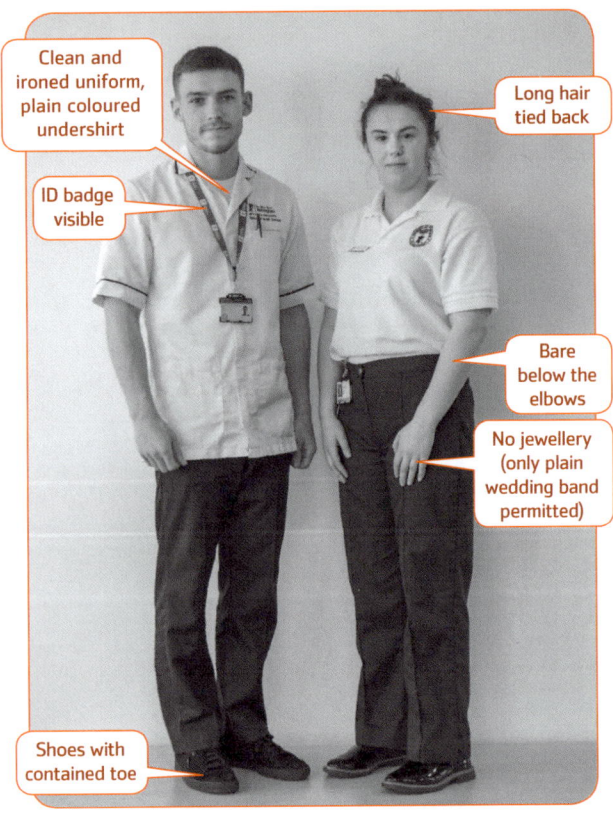

Clean and ironed uniform, plain coloured undershirt

Long hair tied back

ID badge visible

Bare below the elbows

No jewellery (only plain wedding band permitted)

Shoes with contained toe

3   Absence

Make sure you are aware of the absence policy for both your university and your placement area. Usually this means contacting **both areas** if you are unable to attend placement for any reason. This is for your own safety – both areas need to be informed.

It is important that you are certain that you have made contact with your educator before your normal start time. Remember that messages left on voicemail or answerphones may not be picked up. You will need to have contact with your educator to determine how long you may be absent, and when you will be returning to placement. Following local Trust policies, you may have to undertake a return to work assessment once you are well enough to go back to placement.

Top tip

Check the local absence policy, as they may vary across placements. Make a note of relevant contact information in this book.

 Notes

Fill in the tables below:

Placement absence contacts	
Phone number	
Email	
Mobile	

University absence contacts	
Phone number	
Email	
Mobile	

Notes

As a physiotherapy student you have certain responsibilities for both your personal conduct and your professional behaviour as you work towards qualification within a regulated profession. It is important that you understand and engage with these responsibilities during your clinical practice to ensure safety and quality of care.

As a student you are expected to comply with both local policies and the Health and Care Professions Council (HCPC) regulations. Serious breaches of HCPC regulations may mean that you are unable to continue on the course or unable to gain your final qualification / apply for state registration at the end of your studies.

4.1 HCPC guidance on conduct and ethics for students

The HCPC has produced guidance on conduct and ethics for students. In summary it says that students should:

1. Promote and protect the interests of service users and carers
2. Communicate appropriately and effectively
3. Work within the limits of their knowledge and skills
4. Delegate appropriately
5. Respect confidentiality
6. Manage risk
7. Report concerns about safety
8. Be open when things go wrong (this is referred to as duty of candour)
9. Be honest and trustworthy
10. Keep records of their work with service users and carers.

4.2 CSP Code of Professional Values and Behaviours

The Chartered Society of Physiotherapy (CSP) reflects these in its Code of Professional Values and Behaviours that it sets out for its members. The code is built around four key principles:

1. Taking responsibility for your actions
2. Behaving ethically
3. Delivering an effective service
4. Striving to achieve excellence.

> To make it easy for you to access them, we have shortened web links to this format – simply type these into any web browser and you'll go to the right page! Do note that they are case sensitive.

 Activity

Find the HCPC document at bit.ly/HCPC-1 and the CSP document at bit.ly/CSP-Code

Read through them and ensure you understand what is expected of you.

How will your behaviour be different on placement, as compared to being in university?

What does being professional mean to you?

Chartered Society of Physiotherapy (2013) *Code of Members' Professional Values and Behaviour*. CSP.

HCPC (2016) *Guidance on Conduct and Ethics for Students*. HCPC.

Person-centred care (PCC) is a model of care that rejects ideas of healthcare professionals being in positions of power with the patient as a passive recipient of care. PCC ensures that the patient is actively involved in care decisions, placing them at the centre of the team. This approach is considered to be empowering, collaborative, flexible and holistic (based on a biopsychosocial approach). It can be represented by four pillars of care, as shown below. Reflect on this model of care before you begin your placement, and consider what it might mean for your interactions with patients and family.

Exploring the illness/injury experience
Listen to the patient narrative. What are their feelings? What are their ideas? What is their interpretation regarding the impact of illness or injury on function? What are their expectations of treatment, of you and of their role?

Understanding the whole person – consider:
Individual (self-esteem, independence, autonomy, connectedness, spirituality, beliefs)
Family (caregiver burden, disequilibrium)
Socio-environmental context (finance, education/employment, leisure, social support, community)

Finding common ground
Achieve consensus on plan of action for addressing problems/goals
Reflect individual's needs, values and preferences...
...but remain informed by evidence and guidelines

Enhancing the therapeutic relationship
Connect at a human level ("Hello, my name is...")
Demonstrate compassion, empathy and respect
Engender trust

Adapted from:
Stewart, M. *et al.* (2013) *Patient-Centered Medicine: transforming the clinical method*, 3rd edition. Radcliffe Publishing Ltd.

Top tip

You can use a tool to assess how well you are establishing a person-centred approach. The Consultation and Relational Empathy (CARE) measure has been designed for doctors, but applies equally to other healthcare professionals. This tool is free to use, but you should check with your educator first. You can also use it to think about the critical components of communication in a person-centred consultation.

The CARE Measure

© Stewart W. Mercer 2004

1. Please rate the following statements about today's consultation.
Please tick one box for each statement and <u>answer every statement</u>.

How was the doctor at...	Poor	Fair	Good	Very Good	Excellent	Does Not Apply
1. Making you feel at ease....... *(being friendly and warm towards you, treating you with respect; not cold or abrupt)*	☐	☐	☐	☐	☐	☐
2. Letting you tell your "story"....... *(giving you time to fully describe your illness in your own words; not interrupting or diverting you)*	☐	☐	☐	☐	☐	☐
3. Really listening....... *(paying close attention to what you were saying; not looking at the notes or computer as you were talking)*	☐	☐	☐	☐	☐	☐
4. Being interested in you as a whole person... *(asking/knowing relevant details about your life, your situation; not treating you as "just a number")*	☐	☐	☐	☐	☐	☐

(cont'd)

How was the doctor at...	Poor	Fair	Good	Very Good	Excellent	Does Not Apply
5. Fully understanding your concerns....... *(communicating that he/she had accurately understood your concerns; not overlooking or dismissing anything)*	☐	☐	☐	☐	☐	☐
6. Showing care and compassion....... *(seeming genuinely concerned, connecting with you on a human level; not being indifferent or "detached")*	☐	☐	☐	☐	☐	☐
7. Being Positive....... *(having a positive approach and a positive attitude; being honest but not negative about your problems)*	☐	☐	☐	☐	☐	☐
8. Explaining things clearly....... *(fully answering your questions, explaining clearly, giving you adequate information; not being vague)*	☐	☐	☐	☐	☐	☐
9. Helping you to take control....... *(exploring with you what you can do to improve your health yourself; encouraging rather than "lecturing" you)*	☐	☐	☐	☐	☐	☐
10. Making a plan of action with you... *(discussing the options, involving you in decisions as much as you want to be involved; not ignoring your views)*	☐	☐	☐	☐	☐	☐

Reproduced with the kind permission of Dr Stewart Mercer, University of Glasgow.

Mercer, S.W., Watt, G.C.M, Maxwell, M. and Heaney, D.H. (2004) The development and preliminary validation of the Consultation and Relational Empathy (CARE) Measure: an empathy-based consultation process measure. *Family Practice*, **21(6):** 699–705.

As a student on placement you may witness practice that makes you feel uncomfortable and which is not in keeping with the expected professional values. Although you may find it difficult to speak out, you do have a duty of care to your patients and colleagues.

In the first instance speak to your educator, the person in charge of the clinical area or your university support tutor. Both your placement provider and university will have policies on raising concerns that should be easily accessible.

Safeguarding

All staff and students have a duty to safeguard the care and dignity of all healthcare patients. Concerns could relate to a variety of instances such as:

- Alleged abuse of a vulnerable adult or child
- Unsafe or poor practice
- Unethical practice.

Safeguarding training is a mandatory requirement for healthcare professionals. If you have not yet covered this in university you should ask your placement provider if local training is required.

Top tip

Download the **NHS England Safeguarding app** to your phone (available via Apple iOS, Google Play or relevant app store), then you have the relevant information at your fingertips.

7.1 Consent

We must always gain consent before carrying out any intervention. All relevant information must be shared to support individuals in making their own decisions. Consent must be documented according to local policies.

Patients have a right to be informed that you are a student and their wishes respected if they decline treatment.

For consent to be valid:

- It must be given by someone with mental capacity to make the decision
- It has to be voluntary
- Information for the person to understand the pros and cons of receiving the intervention, or not, must be provided.

If a person lacks capacity (for example, if an individual is acutely confused as a result of systemic infection), other people may have to make a decision for them that is deemed to be 'in their best interest'. If you feel that this may be the case during your placement you should seek advice from your supervisor.

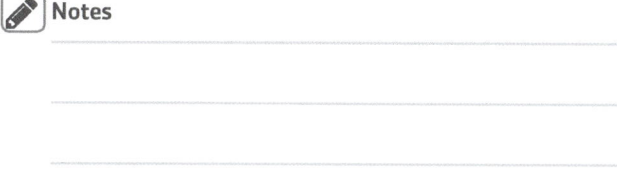

Notes

7.2 Confidentiality

Confidentiality is an integral part of your working practice which your patients, carers and colleagues expect. All patient information must be kept confidential. This includes all written information, any X-rays, images and test results. It should only be shared by those who need to know in order to care for the patient.

As part of your placement you will need to discuss your patients with your supervisor. These conversations need to be done in private – talking while walking down the corridor is not good practice. When having telephone conversations, care needs to be taken that these are not overheard. You may share your placement experiences with your peers but remember that, even though you do not use names, conversations can be overheard by members of the public who may recognise who you are speaking about. Any written reflections or patient case studies that you use in your university work also need to be anonymous.

There is more information for students on the British Medical Association website at bit.ly/BMA-S7

Guidance on social media

Social media can be used to enhance learning and development but needs to be used in a professional manner. Engaging in social media may be an effective way to join in professional debates, find new information and seek out support; however, this needs to be done responsibly.

Tips on using social media responsibly

- Think and pause before you post – how might this affect your professional registration? Remember the HCPC guidance applies both inside and outside work.
- Don't discuss patients, their families or colleagues outside of placement – even if you think you have anonymised them, other people may be able to identify them.
- Do not share anything that may be considered discriminatory or encourages violence or bullying behaviour – always uphold the reputation of the profession.
- Check your privacy settings – others may be able to copy and share your posts more widely.
- Think carefully about what you 'like' or 'retweet', about who and what you associate with or which points of view you support.
- Do not blur professional boundaries with patients by building personal relationships with them – do not 'friend' or 'follow' them online.
- Consider your personal profiles – patients, relations or colleagues may be able to view them online even if you don't engage with them.
- Think about what you may have posted online in the past.

- If you think another student is using social media in a way that is unprofessional or unlawful then you have a duty of care to report your concerns.
- Do not use your mobile phone during working hours unless agreed for work purposes.

> If you are a regular user of social media you should read the CSP guidance document at bit.ly/CSP-SM

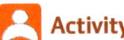 **Activity**

You are about to go on your first placement and your family are keen to keep up to date with how you get on. They are all networked on Instagram and have asked you to post daily pictures and updates from your placement.

What are your considerations in this case?

A few days before your placement, a frequent service user from your placement has found out you are going there and discovered your Twitter profile which states you are a student physiotherapist. They contact you to ask you some questions about their back pain before you start your placement.

What are your actions in this case?

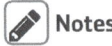 **Notes**

Settling in

As well as becoming oriented to your place of work and getting to know everyone, there are lots of policies and guidelines that you will need to familiarise yourself with. This can be overwhelming so it is good to use the checklist below and make notes.

Orientation

- Staff room, where you can get drinks, eat lunch
- Changing areas and lockers
- Physiotherapy department or ward structure
- Library, study facilities, resources available
- Timetable, hours of work

Policies

- Absence / sickness
- Fire and emergency procedures
- Information governance
- Infection control
- Documentation requirements

Your placement may ask you to provide evidence of mandatory training undertaken in university so make sure you have this to hand:

- Moving and Handling
- Basic Life Support (BLS)
- Infection Control
- Safeguarding
- Information Governance

It is helpful to identify some of the different members of the multidisciplinary team, and also make sure you can distinguish different professions by uniform.

Expectations – working with your educator

It can be hard during your first placement to understand what is expected of you, no matter how well prepared you are. Although there will be some time watching and shadowing your supervisors, you will normally be expected to actively participate. You should expect that your educator will lead and guide you to become more independent, but how this happens will vary across placements and educators.

Your educators will not expect you to know, or be able to do, everything. They will expect you to be honest about what you do not know, and to be willing to have a try. Models of supervision vary widely. You may have one educator or, more commonly, you may have two or more clinicians supervising your work. In some areas two or more students may be supervised by one educator, or it may be that a team model approach is adopted, where a whole team has responsibility for the student(s) placed with it.

Throughout the placement it is important that you ask questions to help you understand what is expected, being as proactive as you can be.

First days of placement

- Share a personal SWOT (see below) with your educator to help them to understand you better; this should include an indication of how you prefer to learn.
- Create some broad objectives about what you would like to achieve while there.
- Discuss these with your educator(s).

- Once you have experienced what your placement might offer you in terms of development, revise your objectives using a SMART framework (see below).
- Agree some formal feedback sessions with your educator – throughout your placement you will receive feedback from your educator on your progress and areas where you could improve. There will also be formal reviews (usually halfway through and at the end) where marks may be awarded and feedback documented. You need to familiarise yourself with any university documentation and marking criteria. Find out if you need to provide your educator with any paperwork or give access to electronic documents.
- Do some preparatory work before review sessions. Consider what's going well and where you need to improve. It is good practice to mark yourself against any criteria which you can compare with your educator's assessment. This promotes discussions around your performance and helps you both make plans to progress.
- You may have visits through your placement from a university tutor. Find out when these will be and check they are scheduled in diaries.
- Make time spent shadowing / observing as active as possible – take notes, ask questions.

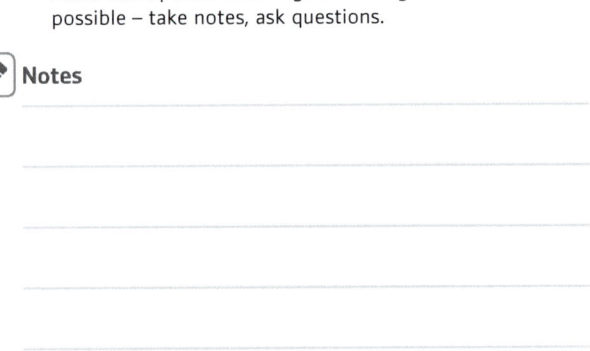 **Notes**

SWOT

SWOT is a simple framework for you to identify your personal qualities. It can be a useful strategic planning tool and to help identify opportunities for development.

Complete the table below and share with your educator.

Strengths	Weaknesses
Opportunities	Threats

Initial objectives	
1	
2	
3	

SMART objectives

By making objectives SMART, they become a useful tool to drive your placement forwards. They help you focus on what you need to do to make incremental progress. They demonstrate to your educator that you are developing and moving forwards. To be most effective they need to be refined and revised throughout the placement. An example of an appropriate objective might be:

'By the end of week one, I can complete a comprehensive subjective assessment'.

SMART stands for

S: specific

M: measurable

A: achievable

R: realistic

T: time bound

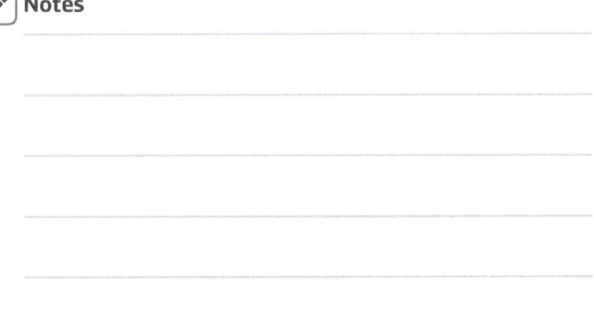 **Notes**

 **Activity**

Read the following account from a student physiotherapist following their first placement.

"I really struggled on my first physiotherapy placement. I had fantastic support and I understood the anatomy, etcetera. But the thing that really bothered me was feeling incompetent. There are situations on placement that university can't prepare you for, whether it be a mystery pain that you can't figure out or a serious condition you've never dealt with before, or whether it simply be a difficult patient. These situations overwhelmed me. I'm used to being 110% prepared for all my exams, lessons and lectures, so going into a situation where I felt thoroughly unprepared and incompetent really threw me, to a point where I actually cried. But the thing you have to be reassured of is that this is normal. You aren't supposed to be prepared for all these situations and that's okay. You are actually meant to go in to them not knowing how to deal with them and not getting it right this time. That's because there is no other way of learning how to deal with it other than via your own experience. Every physio (be it a 3rd year, lecturer, educator) will have been equally as unprepared the first time they encountered this situation – and they will not judge you for how you deal with it. The important thing is that you remember the experience and learn from it."

 Notes

_____

_____

_____

Communicating with patients and carers

Communication is a core physiotherapy skill, which is critical for effective therapeutic interpersonal relationships and person-centred care. Effective communication is associated with significantly improved patient experience and reduced adverse incidents/complaints. It also has benefits for healthcare professionals – reduced stress, greater work satisfaction and improved self-confidence.

Effective communication checklist

✓	Always make a positive connection with your patient and their family. Introduce yourself and state your role, explaining that you are a **student** physiotherapist. Establish how the patient prefers to be addressed.
✓	Pay attention to your own (and the patient's) non-verbal behaviour – make eye contact and assume an open posture. If your patient is sitting or lying, adjust your position so that you are at the same level.
✓	Always explain what you plan to do and why – this will help put the patient at ease, manage expectations and begin the process of informed consent.
✓	Speak clearly and use terminology that is appropriate for your patient. Consider age, understanding, cognitive impairments and level of knowledge.
✓	Consider using open questions to gain more detailed information from patients and carers.
✓	Practise active listening: remove distractions; respond appropriately to the patient's body language; seek clarification where necessary; try paraphrasing/summarising the patient narrative to check your understanding; delay evaluation; maintain attention; listen for content and feelings.

✓	Deliver information in 'chunks' – this avoids overwhelming the patient and causing confusion. Always check that you have been understood, and correct any misunderstandings.
✓	Reflect on your communication, and analyse your strengths and weaknesses. Discuss these with your educator who can help you identify your communication development needs.

Barriers to communication are as follows:

PAIN AND FATIGUE
Prioritise the information needed and return once the patient has had opportunity to sleep or when their pain is better controlled.

FEAR AND ANXIETY
Reassure patients and provide a safe environment for them to discuss their experiences and concerns. Reassure them that there are no 'silly questions'.

TIME
Try to protect time to talk to your patients and minimise interruptions. If you are interrupted explain why you have to leave and when you will return.

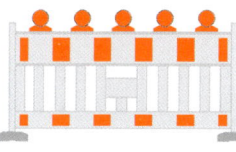

ENVIRONMENT
Reduce background noise where possible, especially if your patient has hearing or cognitive impairments.

LANGUAGE
Avoid slang, jargon and ambiguous terms. Consider help from a translator for patients who are not fluent in English.

VALUES AND BELIEFS
Be aware that people have different sociocultural values and beliefs. Develop cultural competency.

The novice communicator

It is entirely natural to feel nervous when you first start to communicate with patients and relatives in your role as a student physiotherapist. Think of strategies to help you manage your anxieties so that the effectiveness of your communication is not adversely affected, and the patient has confidence in you.

Top tips

- Prepare! Know what you need to say to the patient and the purpose of your interaction.
- Collect any documentation or equipment that you might also need.
- Mentally rehearse the opening to your conversation – feeling fluent and articulate will make you feel more relaxed and put your patient at ease.
- Practise focal relaxation as you approach the patient – try some controlled breathing, push your shoulders down and stretch your hands open.
- There may be opportunity during your placement to spend time talking to patients and their families outside of a treatment setting – these are often opportunities to build your confidence.

Dealing with difficult situations

DO NOT attempt to answer patients' questions if you are not confident of the answer. Be honest with your patient and tell them that you don't know – but make sure you find the person who can deal with the situation.

DO be careful with your non-verbal communication, especially facial expressions. Try not to look shocked or disgusted if confronted with uncomfortable sights or disclosures – this can make your patient feel judged or uncomfortable.

DO remember that whilst family members can be very supportive and helpful, there may be times that you have to ask them to leave the room / area in order to protect patient confidentiality.

DO remember that bad news is any information which adversely affects your patient's view of their future. Using a communication model, such as SPIKES, can help you frame the conversation clearly, honestly and sensitively.

S	**S**etting up the interview: consider where, when, who should be present.
P	Assessing the patient's **P**erception: establish what the patient knows so far.
I	Obtaining the patient's **I**nvitation: find out how much the patient wants to know at this moment.
K	Giving **K**nowledge and information to the patient: diagnosis, treatment plan, prognosis and support.
E	Addressing the patient's **E**motions with empathetic responses: respond to the patient's feelings. Do not try to give further information if the patient is experiencing strong emotional reactions.
S	**S**trategy and **S**ummary: identify coping strategies and other sources of support. Reflect on your own emotions before you move on to your next patient.

Notes

Ali, M. (2017) Communication skills 1: benefits of effective communication for patients. *Nursing Times*, **113(12)**: 18–19.

Baile, W.F. *et al.* (2000) SPIKES – a six-step protocol for delivering bad news: application to the patient with cancer. *The Oncologist*, **5(4)**: 302–11.

HCPC (2013) *Standards of Proficiency for Physiotherapists* (online). Available at: bit.ly/HCPC-2

12 Communicating with the multidisciplinary team

Effective communication between healthcare professionals is a critical factor in achieving good patient outcomes. Miscommunication is implicated in many adverse events and professional conflict. Research suggests that shared training programmes and simulation may be useful methods for enhancing interprofessional communication. Standardised communication tools are also valuable for conveying important information accurately and concisely. A number of organisations, including the World Health Organization, recognise SBAR (Situation, Background, Assessment and Recommendation) as a reliable and validated tool, effective in the promotion of patient safety.

Situation	What is currently happening? – concise statement of the immediate problem
Background	Relevant and brief details of the circumstances leading up to this situation
Assessment	What you have found / what you think the problem is
Recommendation	What is recommended or requested to resolve the problem

 Notes

Example of an SBAR communication between physiotherapist and doctor

S   Hi, this is Jane Beeton, the physiotherapist calling from ward 10. I have just seen Jack Wheeler, a 77-year-old male patient who was admitted 3 days ago with a urinary tract infection, for which he has been receiving intravenous antibiotics. This morning he collapsed whilst mobilising.

B   Jack is normally independently mobile with the aid of a stick. He has osteoarthritis in his left hip, controlled hypertension and type 2 diabetes. This morning we were asked to assess Jack's mobility. After taking a few steps away from the bed, Jack complained of feeling unwell, fainted and we lowered him to the floor. Once help arrived we assisted him back into bed.

A   Jack's observations prior to mobilisation were all stable. Jack lost consciousness for less than 30 seconds. I have completed a further set of observations prior to this call. He is sitting up in bed and talking. His respiratory rate is 12 and he is breathing room air; his oxygen saturations are 97%. Jack's blood pressure is 120/85 mmHg and his heart rate is 105. He is apyrexial. He is alert and oriented and his blood sugar levels are normal. He has sustained a graze and a bruise to his left shoulder but there are no other injuries apparent. I believe that his fall was a result of a postural drop in blood pressure.

R   Please assess this patient with a view to establishing any injuries and also reviewing his blood pressure. I have asked the nurses to continue observations as per the National Early Warning Score (NEWS2) protocol.

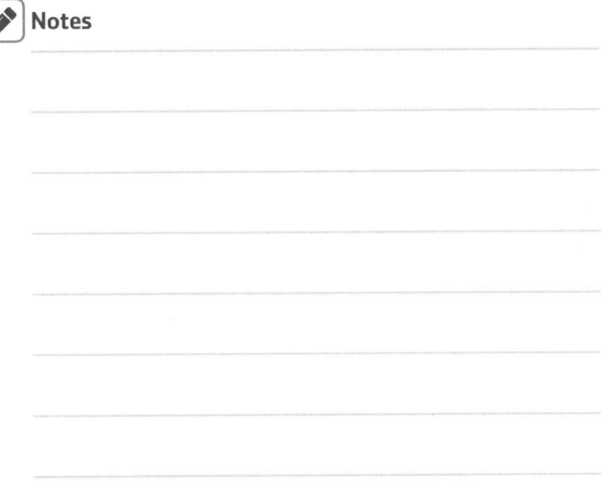

Top tip

Some of the terminology used in clinical practice can be quite perplexing – ask if you do not understand, and keep a list of new words or terms in your notebook for reference.

Whilst participating in multi-professional simulation training may feel quite daunting as a student, remember that these are very valuable learning opportunities to take advantage of. You will receive helpful formative feedback that you can use to reflect upon and further develop your communication skills.

Notes

_____

_____

_____

_____

_____

_____

_____

_____

Foronda, C., MacWilliams, B. and McArthur, E. (2016) Interprofessional communication in healthcare: an integrative review. *Nurse Education in Practice*, **19:** 36–40.

Being there

Healthcare-associated infection is a significant problem causing potentially serious illness, long-term disability and death. The financial and emotional cost of these infections is considerable. Most of these infections are, however, preventable; as such, you have a responsibility to yourself, your patients and your colleagues to comply with national and local guidance.

Hand washing is a fundamental component of infection control – you must wash your hands before and after every patient contact, including contact with the patient environment.

Notes

RUB HANDS FOR HAND HYGIENE! WASH HANDS WHEN VISIBLY SOILED

⏱ **Duration of the entire procedure: 20-30 seconds**

1a 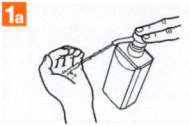 **1b** 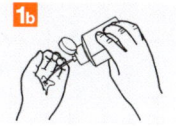 **2**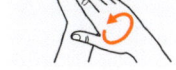

Apply a palmful of the product in a cupped hand, covering all surfaces;

Rub hands palm to palm;

3 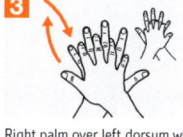 **4** **5**

Right palm over left dorsum with interlaced fingers and vice versa;

Palm to palm with fingers interlaced;

Backs of fingers to opposing palms with fingers interlocked;

6 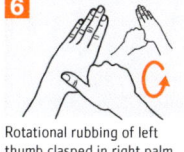 **7** 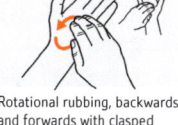 **8**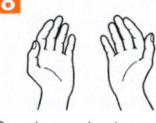

Rotational rubbing of left thumb clasped in right palm and vice versa;

Rotational rubbing, backwards and forwards with clasped fingers of right hand in left palm and vice versa;

Once dry, your hands are safe.

Proper hand rub technique (World Health Organization, 2009). Reproduced with permission of the World Health Organization, www.who.int.

Directions for hand washing (World Health Organization, 2009):

- Wet hands with water
- Apply soap
- Rub hands together (palm to palm)
- Interlock fingers, alternating hands (palm to palm and top of hand to palm)

- Back of fingers to opposing palms with fingers interlocked
- Rub each thumb thoroughly
- Circular motion of fingertips in opposite palm
- Rinse hands with water
- Dry hands thoroughly with a single-use paper towel
- Use towel or elbows to turn off taps

In certain situations you may be required to wear personal protective equipment (PPE). This may include disposable gloves, aprons, eye protectors or face masks. You should follow the instructions on the signage in your local working area. If you are unsure ask a member of staff or your educator – do not make assumptions.

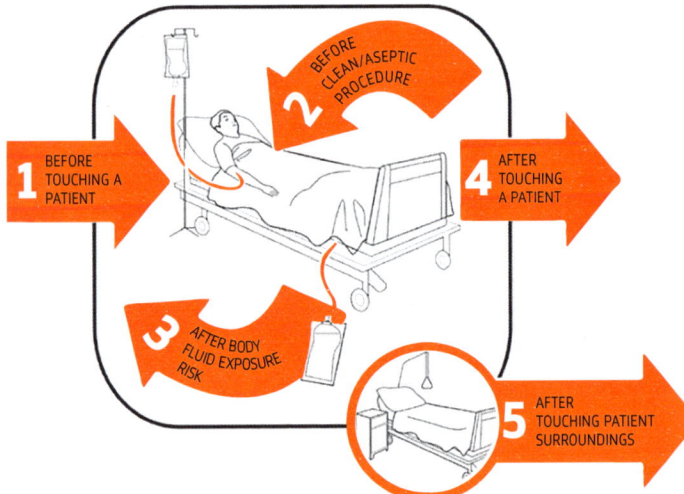

1 BEFORE TOUCHING A PATIENT

2 BEFORE CLEAN/ASEPTIC PROCEDURE

3 AFTER BODY FLUID EXPOSURE RISK

4 AFTER TOUCHING A PATIENT

5 AFTER TOUCHING PATIENT SURROUNDINGS

My Five Moments for hand hygiene. Reprinted from *Journal of Hospital Infection*, 67(1), Sax, H. *et al.*, 'My five moments for hand hygiene': a user-centred design approach to understand, train, monitor and report hand hygiene, pp. 9–21 (2007), with permission from Elsevier.

Placement is time to put all the theory and principles you have learnt about moving and handling into practice. Real-life situations can be challenging – working in a dynamic environment and with patients who may be in pain and have limited mobility. You will also be expected to work alongside other staff who may expect you to take the lead as they often regard physiotherapists as knowledgeable in this field. You may also be asked to advise other healthcare professionals about the safest way to move or mobilise patients.

It is essential that approved techniques are used to protect both patients and yourself from injury.

14.1 Assessing risk with TILE

Before carrying out **any** manual handling task, whether this involves moving a patient or a piece of equipment, you must assess the risk.

Task	What do you want to do / achieve?
Individual	What are your individual capabilities? Consider your own health and ability – do you have any injuries or health conditions? Consider the abilities of other colleagues involved.
Load	This refers to the patient or object. Additional equipment may be necessary.
Environment	Consider the space / environment that you are working in – you may have to remove potential hazards, check patients' footwear, attend to drips and drains.

Common tasks you may come across

- Getting a patient out of bed, or moving them in the bed
- Assisting the patient on / off toilet / commode
- Teaching a patient to use a walking stick / frame / crutches
- Using patients' aids such as a standing aid, sliding sheet or hoist (check local policies or guidelines).

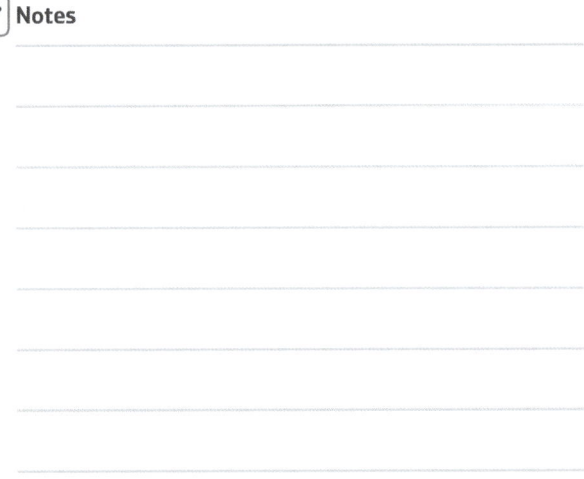

Top tip

Before going out on placement:

- Revise how to measure for correct height of sticks, frame and crutches
- Practise teaching gait patterns (including stair ascent / descent).

Notes

The most common form of notes used by physiotherapists, in a variety of settings, is SOAP (Subjective, Objective, Analysis, Plan) notes. During placement you will have opportunity to develop your note-writing skills, so you should be familiar with the SOAP framework.

There are also many other forms of important documentation that may be useful to look at whilst you are on placement. For example, if you are in a ward-based setting it will be relevant to look at a patient's drug and observation charts, as well as nursing and medical notes. If you need to write in the medical notes, you can still use the SOAP format to frame your documentation. Ask your educator to signpost you to important documentation sources. Do remember that some placements will use electronic records.

🖉 **Notes**

S: Subjective

Always document that you have received consent.

	Could include:
History of present condition (HPC)	Onset – traumatic, insidious, post-surgery Are you the first health professional seen? Previous investigations and treatments Getting better or worse
Present condition (PC)	What are the primary concerns / symptoms, e.g. pain, breathlessness, fatigue, function? Interrogate symptoms (consider use of SOCRATES; see *Chapter 19*) Red Flag questions where relevant
Past medical history (PMH)	*Think THREADS + M* **T**hyroid **H**eart and circulatory system **R**A/OA and bone diseases **E**pilepsy or other neurological conditions **A**sthma or other respiratory conditions **D**iabetes **S**urgery, cancer history, injections **M**ental health issues
Drug history (DH)	What medications are they on, how often do they take them and how?
Social history (SH)	Family / home life. Occupation past or present. Type of work. Activities / hobbies / sports
Physical activity history	Consider physical activity as a vital sign – ask patients about their current level of activity, and establish whether they meet the Chief Medical Officer recommendations. If they do not, ask if they would like advice on increasing their activity levels, in line with Making Every Contact Count
Beliefs, expectations and goals (BEG)	What do they believe is causing their pain or other symptoms? What are their expectations of physio? What are their goals?

O: Objective

In the objective section of the SOAP notes you record the findings of objectively measured tests. In a musculoskeletal setting, for example, this could include the following:

- Observation
- Palpation
- Active and passive range of motion
- Muscle testing – length and strength
- Relevant vital signs, e.g. blood pressure and heart rate
- Special tests
- Neural assessment if indicated
- What treatments you attempted (if relevant).

A: Analysis

The first line of the analysis should always indicate the primary hypothesis based upon the findings of the subjective and objective assessments – a problem list could be included here. For follow-up assessments, the analysis should also detail response to treatment intervention.

P: Plan

Your plan should indicate when the next treatment session will be scheduled. It should also include a treatment plan which links to the problem list and patient goals. The treatment plan should be written using SMART objectives (see *Chapter 10*).

Why is good note-keeping so important?

- It reminds you of your patients' issues, problem lists and what further treatments you are going to attempt in future sessions.
- In the extremely rare instances of a patient's case being reviewed for medico-legal reasons, you can show that you

have completed your role safely, and assessed and treated the patient to a professional standard.

- It allows other healthcare professionals to understand your management approach, and continue if necessary.
- For the benefit of audit, service evaluation and quality improvement.
- Remember that all student notes need countersigning by a qualified healthcare professional.

✏️ Notes

16.1 Ward-based placements

Ward-based placements may be extremely diverse, and are excellent environments for practising and developing your skills. Remember that while the ward may be aligned to a particular speciality (for example trauma orthopaedics), the likelihood is that you will encounter many different types of patients (for example, those with co-existing respiratory or neurological conditions).

What might a typical day look like?

8:00 – 8:30	**Physio department morning meeting** – The whole of the departmental team meets for any important announcements and to plan for the day.
9:00 – 9:45	**Ward round** – The ward round is a meeting of all healthcare professionals on the ward. Doctors, nurses, physios, occupational therapists (OTs), discharge coordinators and any other healthcare professionals may be present. During the meeting, every patient on the ward will be briefly discussed with regard to their medical management plan, any tasks needing to be completed and their discharge plan.
9:45 – 12:00	**Seeing patients** – During the morning your educator will have prioritised the patients you need to see that day. In the morning you will see the higher priority patients. As you develop through the placement, prioritisation of patients is likely to become your responsibility.

12:00 – 13:00	**Lunch** – Many wards have protected mealtimes for their patients, during which time it is advised that they have no interventions from physiotherapy unless absolutely necessary. This is a good time to take your own lunch!
13:00 – 16:00	**Seeing patients** – During the afternoon you may review patients who require a second treatment, as well as the lower priority patients.

Before seeing a patient

1. Read through patient notes. Things to look for include:
   - Reason for admission (i.e. their presenting condition) and date of admission
   - Any surgery/intervention undertaken, and related post-op/post-intervention medical instructions with regard to weight-bearing or mobility status
   - Pathway of the patient – where have they been admitted from (e.g. other wards, A&E, home)?
   - Past medical history – ensure that the patient has no contraindications or precautions to your planned treatment
   - Social history – where does the patient live? A care home or their own home? Who do they live with? Do they live in a bungalow or house (which will be relevant if they then need to practise stairs before discharge)? How do they normally mobilise? What is their occupation?
   - Be aware of their current medical plan from the medical notes
   - If previously seen by physiotherapy, what were the findings and interventions?
2. Ensure the patient is medically stable and well enough for physiotherapy. Check their observations and National Early Warning Score (NEWS2) (see inside back cover).

3. Speak to the patient's named nurse (or the nurse in charge), asking how the patient has been during the day. Have they been out of bed and mobilised, and if so, how? It is often helpful to ask if the patient has had any required medications, e.g. analgesia or bronchodilators.

4. Collect any equipment necessary to mobilise the patient (e.g. hoists, sliding sheets, frames, walking sticks, etc.).

Seeing a patient

Introduce yourself to your patient and conduct a subjective and objective assessment. Be aware that you might be mobilising a patient who has been in bed for some time, so consider issues such as fatigue, orthostatic intolerance (postural drops in blood pressure) and breathlessness. Make sure the environment is safe and free of clutter.

After seeing a patient

After treating a patient, it is important that you leave them comfortable, well supported and with any necessary items within reach, e.g. the nurse call buzzer, a drink (as long as the patient is not nil by mouth), or the patient-controlled analgesia handset. It is good practice to ask if there is anything else you can do for them before you leave.

Document all assessment findings and treatment interventions in the MDT notes. You must get these notes countersigned by your educator. Inform the doctors and nurses of anything relevant that occurred during your interaction; this may be important for the ongoing medical plan or if there are positioning or observation requirements that the nurses will need to attend to.

Consider relevant outcome measures

The choice of outcome measures may be influenced by many factors including use of NHS Trust specific measures, or educator preferred measures. It is helpful to speak to your educator for guidance. Some commonly used outcome measures in a ward setting may include:

- Tinetti Test – a test for balance and gait
- Elderly Mobility Scale – a measure of global mobility
- Timed Up and Go Test – a mobility measure
- Timed Up and Supported Steady Stand – a measure of standing balance
- Vital signs – assess physiological stability.

ℹ️ Top tip

A ward-based placement is a fantastic way to experience the whole MDT in action. Talk to other members of the team on your ward. If there is time available ask to shadow another healthcare professional. Observing an OT or Speech and Language Therapy assessment can give you a different perspective on patients' needs as well as developing your knowledge of other professional roles.

ALWAYS get your notes countersigned by your educator.

Be confident, but never be afraid to ask a question. Checking with your educator (or other qualified healthcare professional) not only develops your knowledge, but can also prevent serious safety issues.

What if I'm asked to treat a patient with a respiratory problem?

On a general medical or surgical ward it is very likely that some of the patients will be referred to physiotherapy for respiratory management. It is important to consider how their medical condition will influence your interventions.

Respiratory subjective assessment

A respiratory subjective assessment focuses on five cardinal symptoms.

1. Breathlessness (consider descriptors and use of a visual analogue scale or Borg scale, and impact on exercise tolerance)
2. Cough
3. Sputum
4. Wheeze
5. Pain (see *Chapter 19: Pain assessment*)

For each of these symptoms you may wish to ask about a 24-hour pattern, aggravating and easing factors and other more specific questions. For example, with sputum production, you may want to ask about amount, colour and viscosity. It is also important to ascertain whether the current state represents a change for the patient and if so, how?

Respiratory objective assessment

Objective assessment includes observation of the patient's breathing pattern, colour and use of supplemental oxygen. You will also need to interpret vital signs, arterial blood gases or chest X-rays. You may be required to auscultate (listen to breath sounds), palpate the patient's chest, as well as perform some simple spirometry. If you have yet to cover a respiratory module, your educator will be happy to demonstrate these techniques to you.

 Notes

Respiratory management

Respiratory management is broadly aimed at addressing the following problems:

- Decreased lung volumes
- Increased work of breathing
- Decreased exercise tolerance
- Inability to clear secretions.

ℹ An example

You are on a ward-based placement, about to see patient A. In their notes you notice a history of chronic obstructive pulmonary disease (COPD). When observing the patient you notice that they have a high respiratory rate and they are complaining of breathlessness.

On assessment, the patient has oxygen saturations of 85% (previously 94% whilst breathing room air). On auscultating (listening to) their chest, you hear breath sounds throughout, but with added coarse crackles. You are aware that this may indicate the presence of retained secretions. Despite multiple attempts to get the patient to cough and expectorate the secretions, they are unable to do so.

You plan to assist the patient to clear secretions (for example use of nebulisers, positioning and Active Cycle of Breathing techniques). You speak to your educator and nurse in charge about the patient – a decision is made to start some oxygen therapy. These actions restore the patient's oxygen saturations to target levels, and reduce their work of breathing, respiratory rate and breathlessness.

Main, E. & Denehy, L. (2016) *Cardiorespiratory Physiotherapy: adults and paediatrics*, 5th edition. Elsevier.

What if I'm asked to treat a patient with a neurological problem?

Even during your early placements you may be asked to see patients with neurological conditions such as stroke, Parkinson's disease, multiple sclerosis (MS), motor neurone disease (MND) or traumatic brain injury. It is important to consider how these conditions might influence your approach to assessment.

Neurological subjective assessment

Neurological assessments can be very complex and are often multi-faceted. In the first instance, try to keep your approach simple and functional. In addition to the usual subjective assessment it may be helpful to consider:

- Nature and stage of the disease/injury – for example, is this an acute or chronic presentation? Is it a progressive condition? These factors will have implications for rehabilitation and goal setting
- Function and mobility – falls history
- Presenting complaints – what is their primary complaint? Weakness, decreased ROM, tonal issues, sensation, proprioception, balance, coordination? Relate all these factors back to function
- Previous treatments
- Social and home factors – is their home adapted?

Do remember that speech and swallowing may be affected in patients with neurological conditions, as well as cognition, concentration and ability to follow commands.

Neurological objective assessment

A good tip is to keep your objective assessment functional. Observe the patient completing a task that is important to them such as:

- Sit to stand for a pivot transfer from wheelchair to toilet seat

- Gait
- Reach to grasp.

Break down these tasks to analyse the expected movements at each joint level. If there is a kinematic abnormality, consider the cause – is it weakness, or a tonal or proprioceptive issue? Once this has been identified you can investigate in more detail.

In some instances, it may not be possible to assess in this way. You may encounter patients whose functional level is so low, as a result of a neurological condition or injury, that they lie in bed most of the day and transfer via a hoist. In these cases, the physiotherapy focus may include positioning (to maintain skin integrity and limit contractures), assisted transfers (to mitigate the adverse effects of bed rest) and potentially the treatment of any respiratory complications.

Neurological treatment

Once the primary cause of the kinematic abnormality has been identified you can plan how to treat this through interventions such as exercise, resistance/strength training and stretching. Base your treatment on functional activity in order to improve patient engagement. Remember to use appropriate outcome measures to track the patient's progress.

Key training components to consider in neurological practice:

- Feedback (knowledge of results/performance, internal and external, concurrent, summary or faded)
- Instructions (specific and brief)
- Progression/challenging the patient
- Number of sets and repetitions
- Functional/task-specific
- Random practice/variable practice (initially block practice)
- Bimanual and unilateral activities

- Outcome measures
- High intensity of meaningful exercises
- External cues / external focus for feedback
- Closed chain exercises in lower limb
- Active participation
- Mental practice

 **Example**

Patient B suffered a left-sided stroke one month ago. He has decreased dorsiflexion at his right ankle while walking. Functionally this means he is continually tripping over his right foot and has a significant history of falls.

In your clinical reasoning you consider that this issue could be due to weakness of his dorsiflexors, such as tibialis anterior, or tightness of the antagonist plantarflexors. It may also be a tonal issue with potentially high tone in his plantarflexors limiting ankle dorsiflexion.

You choose to assess:

- Strength of ankle dorsiflexors using the MRC scale
- Passive vs. active ankle dorsiflexion ROM
- For tone of plantarflexors by an ankle-jerk test
- Lower limb sensation.

Notes

Carr, J. & Shepherd, R. (2003) *Stroke Rehabilitation – guidelines for exercise and training to optimize motor skill.* Butterworth-Heinemann.

16.2 Musculoskeletal outpatients

Your first musculoskeletal outpatients (MSK OP) placement provides the opportunity to practise the assessment and treatment skills that you have learnt in the classroom, as well as developing your time management skills. It is very important to remember that some of the patients you see might not have been triaged or assessed by another healthcare professional. Therefore, it is even more critical that you screen for more serious pathologies (consider your red flags; see *Section 16.4*).

What might a typical day look like?

8:00 – 8:30	**Morning meeting or administration time before starting patient list** – During this time, it is advisable to get out all of the notes and/or referrals for your patients for the rest of the day. Have a quick look through any new referrals and plan your day.
9:00 – 12:30	**Seeing patients** – On your first MSK OP placement, your educator may initially sit in on your consultations, but gradually you should progress to being more independent in your practice. You might have time blocked out after each patient you have seen to write notes and discuss the case with your educator. However, this might not always be possible and you may have limited time for note-keeping. In these instances, it is advisable to jot down a couple of the key assessment findings so that, when you come back to the notes later, you can remember what you did.
12:30 – 13:00	**Lunch** – Lunch times will not always be fixed on these placements; you will have to get used to being flexible.
13:00 – 16:00	**Seeing patients** – As morning.

Plan

MSK OP placements often involve very busy, fast-paced days; you can see a large variety and quantity of patients in the course of one day. It is advisable to plan accordingly. When you arrive in the morning, take a look at all of the patients you have listed for that day. In particular, read through any new referrals. The referral should (at the very least) indicate the anatomical region of the pain – however, be aware that some referrals may be incorrect. Despite this, if you know the region, you can start to think about some of the key assessments you may wish to include. Some educators may allow you a crib sheet (concise notes that you can use for quick reference) on your first placement, but discuss this with them first.

Subjective and objective assessment

A standardised subjective and objective assessment is detailed in the SOAP Notes section in this book (see *Chapter 15*). Do remember – this is an example of a basic assessment, and other tests may need to be included.

Time-keeping

The time you are allocated for patients will depend on the working practice of your department. It can vary between 30 minutes per patient to an hour for a first assessment. A realistic goal to set yourself for your first MSK OP placement is to be able to complete a full assessment and have delivered some form of treatment within your allocated timeframe. This won't be easy at first! However, as you develop your subjective and objective assessment skills, and you begin to prioritise what must be included in the current assessment, you will become more efficient. Plan the time you have according to the goals you want to achieve. Your educator can help you with this. It is a good idea to ensure you have a way of telling the time too. A watch next to the patient notes, or a vibrate alarm on your mobile phone in your pocket, could help – ask your educator what they think is appropriate.

Learning to write assessment notes while taking a subjective history is a vital skill that you will develop in time. As with all skills, it takes practice. It can help to have a sheet with pre-prepared headings so that you can fill in the detail as you go.

i Top tip

Always plan the assessment:

What MUST, SHOULD and COULD I assess?

Treat the patient in front of you

Always consider the SIN factors of the patient that you are assessing. What is the **S**everity, **I**rritability and **N**ature of their pain? You can establish this using the SOCRATES mnemonic (see *Chapter 19*). Understanding SIN factors is important as it will influence what you do during your assessment. For example, you may be reviewing a patient whose assessment reveals that their pain is highly irritable. It would then be unwise to undertake many of the (aggravating) special tests which could provoke their symptoms. This could lead to false positives which adversely affect your clinical reasoning. It could also have a negative impact on your therapeutic relationship with the patient, and their compliance with treatment.

A number of your patients may present with acute soft tissue injuries – it is helpful to revise soft tissue injury management before your placement. An acronym like PEACE & LOVE prompts you to think of relevant factors.

P **PROTECTION**
Avoid activities and movements that increase pain during the first few days after injury.

E **ELEVATION**
Elevate the injured limb higher than the heart as often as possible.

A **AVOID ANTI-INFLAMMATORIES**
Avoid taking anti-inflammatory medications as they reduce tissue healing. Avoid icing.

C **COMPRESSION**
Use elastic bandage or taping to reduce swelling.

E **EDUCATION**
Your body knows best. Avoid unnecessary passive treatments and medical investigations and let nature play its role.

&

L **LOAD**
Let pain guide your gradual return to normal activities. Your body will tell you when it's safe to increase load.

O **OPTIMISM**
Condition your brain for optimal recovery by being confident and positive.

V **VASCULARISATION**
Choose pain-free cardiovascular activities to increase blood flow to repairing tissues.

E **EXERCISE**
Restore mobility, strength and proprioception by adopting an active approach to recovery.

Reproduced with the kind permission of Blaise Dubois, The Running Clinic.

Dubois, B. & Esculier, J-F. (2019) Soft tissue injuries simply need PEACE & LOVE. *British Journal of Sports Medicine* blog. Available at: bit.ly/MSK-PL

Use your 'free' time well – it is not uncommon to have half an hour to an hour between sessions with patients. Plan an assessment for your next patient, finish your notes and/or discuss your previous patient with your educator. You might also ask to observe one of the other physiotherapists in the team – this is a great way to learn about other approaches and perspectives.

'Embrace the grey' – not everything in the clinical world is clear-cut. For example, on placement you may experience patients who are in persistent or chronic pain. These patients can be very complex and it can be difficult to explain or clinically reason all of your findings. You should aim to be comfortable with some ambiguity, but discuss with your educator to ensure that you have not missed anything significant.

Do not be alarmed if you are unsure of a patient's condition – sometimes it can take two or three sessions to build up a comprehensive picture and be able to make an informed clinical diagnosis.

16.3 Community placements

Community placements offer physiotherapy students a range of experiences and conditions, with the added challenge of delivering assessment and treatment within the homes of patients, or in care homes. In the community setting it is likely that you will encounter elderly patients who have a number of co-morbidities that could span neurological, respiratory and/or musculoskeletal domains, as well as other specialist areas. Mobility is key; assessing patients' needs and providing them with equipment to aid their mobility and improve compliance with physical activity guidelines will be your primary role.

Importantly, however, a community placement requires you to think on your feet. In the domiciliary environment you often do not have access to traditional exercise equipment and therefore you will need to be creative in devising useful, functional alternatives.

What might a typical day look like?

8:00 – 9:00	**Morning meeting** – In the community therapy team, it is likely that there will be nurses, OTs and potentially other professionals too. A morning meeting will often take place to discuss the patients to be seen that day and to decide if joint assessments / treatment sessions are required. Patient triage may also occur during these meetings.
9:00 – 12:00	**Seeing patients** – The advantages of community sessions are that you will often spend a significant amount of time with your patients. Travelling to their homes / care homes gives you ample opportunity to assess and treat them in their own environment.
12:00 – 13:00	**Lunch** – May be on the move – make sure you take a packed lunch!
13:00 – 16:00	**Seeing patients** – As above

Multidisciplinary team working

Community placements will expose you to significant MDT working. Often you will be expected to carry out many roles that you may have previously considered as primarily nursing or OT roles; for example, calculating Waterlow Scores (to assess the risk of pressure ulcers) and completing skin assessments. Joint assessments are common and where these are not possible, an OT or nurse may instruct you to complete an assessment or task on their behalf when you go out to see a patient. Become comfortable with a blurring of professional boundaries when it comes to roles and responsibilities, but always ensure that you feel competent and confident with what you are doing. If you are unsure, ask your educator for guidance or assistance.

Respecting patients' homes

As student healthcare professionals you should consider it a privilege to be allowed inside patients' homes. Consider how you might feel if someone came into your house and did not treat your home, belongings and yourself/family with respect, dignity and cultural competency. Think very carefully about your actions. As you will be working in patients' homes, and at a distance from your base, it is also important that safety precautions are adhered to. For example, there may be a calling or messaging system that you should familiarise yourself with on the first day.

ℹ️ Top tip

Function is key! Assessing patients in their own homes gives you the perfect opportunity to see how they transfer, mobilise or complete functional activities in the domiciliary context. These activities can look very different compared to the clinical context of a hospital or rehabilitation unit! Seeing how patients manage activities of daily living can help you to assess where additional services, an aid or appliance, or other physiotherapy input (such as exercise therapy) may be indicated to improve safety and/or function.

16.4 Red Flags – indicators for serious pathology

Many healthcare professionals use a flag system to help indicate various clinical and psychosocial issues that may be of use in terms of diagnosis, assessment and planning:

Red	• Indicators of serious pathology or biomedical factors
Orange	• Indicators of psychiatric symptoms: • Clinical depression, generalised anxiety disorder

Yellow	• Psychological factors that may impact prognosis:
	  • Beliefs and behaviours
	  • Emotions
	  • Willingness to change

Blue	• Occupational beliefs that may impact prognosis: • Belief that work will cause injury

Black	• Socio-occupational factors that may impact prognosis:
	  • Work satisfaction
	  • Litigation
	  • Health benefits
	  • Family impact

Red Flags are important questions that you should consider – especially in MSK OP settings, where you could be the first healthcare professional assessing the patient for that particular complaint. However, even on wards and in the community you should remain mindful of concerning symptoms.

Serious pathology	Red Flag questions
Cauda equina syndrome	Saddle anaesthesia?
	Bladder and bowel dysfunction – specifically urinary retention and faecal incontinence?
	Gait disturbance?
	Radicular pain in the legs?
	Bilateral neural symptoms?
Fractures	Trauma?
	May also be prudent to assess for bone density risk factors such as age, post-menopausal women, osteoporosis, long-term steroid user, activity levels during teenage years?
Cancer	Previous history of cancer?
	Generally unwell?
	Unexplained weight loss?
	Failure to respond to normal treatment?
Infection	Night pain?
	Fever?
	Night sweats?
	Generally unwell?
	Tuberculosis? HIV? Rheumatoid arthritis?
	Intravenous drug abuser?
	On immunosuppressant drugs?
DVT (deep vein thrombosis)	DVT Wells' score (NICE, 2015) – an estimate of probability of DVT

Sometimes, one or two of the questions may exhibit a positive answer but should not be considered threatening by themselves. For example, someone with a common mechanical musculoskeletal condition may have night pain, but that finding in isolation should not be considered an alarming factor. Some studies suggest 80% of low back pain patients may have at least one positive Red Flag answer (Underwood, 2009). It is imperative that you link the responses with the clinical picture in front of you. If you are unsure of the significance of a positive finding, always consult with your educator.

It is a good idea to plan how you will ask some of the Red Flag questions. For example, when asking about saddle anaesthesia, you may have to phrase it as "can you feel it when you wipe yourself after going to the toilet?" Get comfortable with asking these questions – they should become part of your repertoire.

16.5 Clinical reasoning

On your early placements, you will usually be asked to take patients' subjective histories and formulate a working diagnosis for discussion with your educator. The following algorithm can be used to help guide you in this process. This is referred to as clinical reasoning which means the logical development of your thoughts about what the problem is, in collaboration with your patient, and using a variety of findings and information sources.

NICE (2015) *Venous thromboembolic diseases: diagnosis, management and thrombophilia testing.* Available at: bit.ly/CG-144

Nicholas, M.K., Linton, S.J., Watson, P.J. and Main, C.J. (2011) Early identification and management of psychological risk factors ("yellow flags") in patients with low back pain: a reappraisal. *Physical Therapy*, **91**: 737–53.

Underwood, M. (2009) Diagnosing acute nonspecific low back pain: time to lower the red flags? *Arthritis & Rheumatism*, **60**: 2855–7.

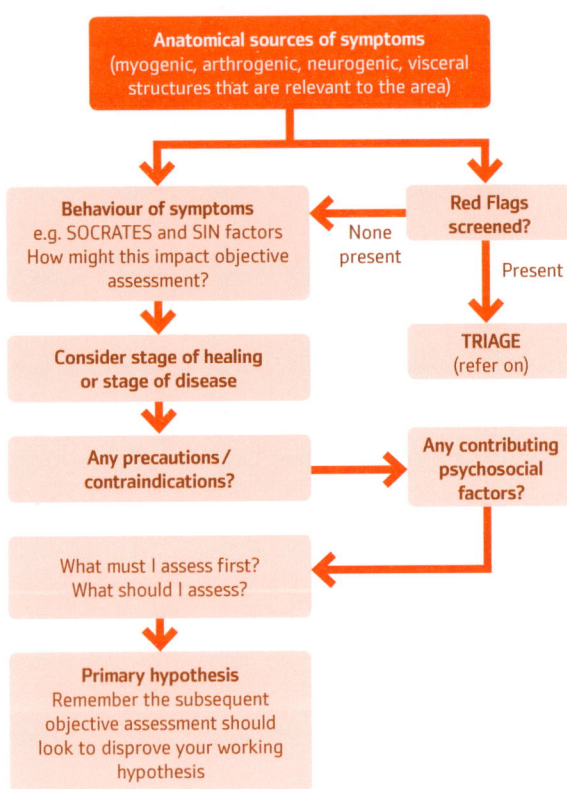

Anatomical sources of symptoms
(myogenic, arthrogenic, neurogenic, visceral structures that are relevant to the area)

Behaviour of symptoms
e.g. SOCRATES and SIN factors
How might this impact objective assessment?

None present

Red Flags screened?

Present

TRIAGE
(refer on)

Consider stage of healing or stage of disease

Any precautions / contraindications?

Any contributing psychosocial factors?

What must I assess first?
What should I assess?

Primary hypothesis
Remember the subsequent objective assessment should look to disprove your working hypothesis

17.1 Basic Life Support (BLS)

If you come across an unresponsive or choking patient in your clinical placement remember to shout for help and that you are never alone. Assess the situation for your own safety first and then intervene. Never do anything that you are not confident of or that puts your own safety at risk.

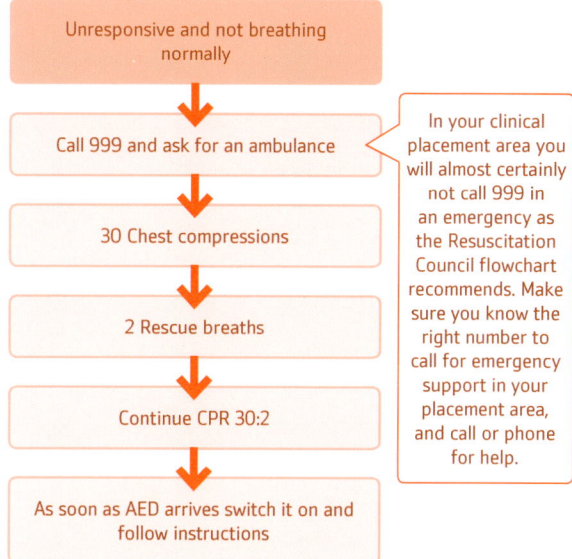

Unresponsive and not breathing normally

Call 999 and ask for an ambulance

30 Chest compressions

2 Rescue breaths

Continue CPR 30:2

As soon as AED arrives switch it on and follow instructions

In your clinical placement area you will almost certainly not call 999 in an emergency as the Resuscitation Council flowchart recommends. Make sure you know the right number to call for emergency support in your placement area, and call or phone for help.

Adult Basic Life Support (Resuscitation Council, 2015).
CPR 30:2 – an emergency cardiopulmonary resuscitation procedure that alternates 30 chest compressions with two rescue breaths; AED – automated external defibrillator (a portable device that checks the heart rhythm and can send an electric shock to the heart to try to restore a normal rhythm). Reproduced with the kind permission of the Resuscitation Council (UK).

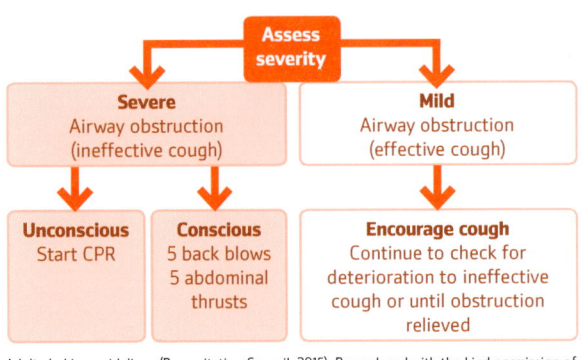

Assess severity

Severe
Airway obstruction
(ineffective cough)

Mild
Airway obstruction
(effective cough)

Unconscious
Start CPR

Conscious
5 back blows
5 abdominal
thrusts

Encourage cough
Continue to check for
deterioration to ineffective
cough or until obstruction
relieved

Adult choking guidelines (Resuscitation Council, 2015). Reproduced with the kind permission of
the Resuscitation Council (UK).

If you need to start CPR see the Adult Basic Life Support
algorithm on the previous page.

- Always keep the
  airway opened by
  tilting the head back
  (head tilt, chin lift).
- Do not put anything
  in the patient's mouth.
- Wait for help before
  moving the patient.
- If it is safe to do so, or
  no neck injury is apparent,
  place in the recovery
  position.
- Time and record events as they
  happen.

The recovery position. Reproduced from *Clinical Skills for
OSCEs*, 5th ed. © Neel Burton, 2015.

Resuscitation Council (2015) Resuscitation guidelines. Available
at: bit.ly/PGCP-7

17.2 ABCDE assessment

There are occasions where you might be involved with patients who have become acutely unwell. Acute physiological deterioration can occur for many reasons including infection, neurological insult, acute cardiac event, electrolyte disturbance, drug reaction, etc.

Physiological 'track and trigger' systems such as NEWS2 (see inside back cover) help healthcare professionals to identify a patient who is deteriorating. Patients' observations are used to create an aggregate score that then allows the team to make decisions regarding monitoring and management. Six simple physiological parameters form the basis of the scoring system:

1. Respiration rate
2. Oxygen saturation
3. Systolic blood pressure
4. Pulse rate
5. Level of consciousness or new confusion
6. Temperature.

It is imperative that you seek help if you are the first person to identify an acutely ill patient. It is helpful to remember the ABCDE acronym to guide your assessment. Normal values can be found on the inside front cover of this book.

Resuscitation Council UK (2019) *The ABCDE Approach*. Available at: bit.ly/RC-ABCDE

Royal College of Physicians (2017) *National Early Warning Score (NEWS2) 2: Standardising the assessment of acute-illness severity in the NHS*. Updated report of a working party. London: RCP, 2017. Available at: bit.ly/NEWS-2

Airway	Check for airway patency – is the patient talking? Can you feel airflow? Are there signs of stridor or cyanosis? If you have concerns about the patient's airway patency shout for help and aim to secure the airway by using the head tilt, chin life manoeuvre. Consider an artificial airway if necessary, and high concentration oxygen therapy.
Breathing	Check respiratory rate, respiratory pattern and oxygen saturations (SpO_2). Auscultate the chest – can you hear breath sounds throughout? Are there added sounds audible? Palpate the chest – can you feel symmetrical movement of the chest wall? Consider supplemental oxygen therapy if necessary. **NB Respiratory rate changes are very sensitive indicators of physiological deterioration. Respiratory rate should be measured accurately – observe and count the patient's breaths over a full minute.**
Circulation	Check blood pressure, heart rate and temperature. Is the patient passing urine? (check fluid balance charts if available). Palpate the radial pulse – is it regular and strong or irregular and weak? Do the extremities look blue or mottled? Do they feel cold to the touch?
Disability	Is the patient alert and oriented? Use the acronym ACVPU (**A**lert, **C**onfused, responds to **V**oice/touch, responds to **P**ain, **U**nresponsive). Are pupils an equal size and do they react to light? Ask a nurse to check the patient's blood sugar levels to exclude hypoglycaemia.
Exposure	Head to toe check – are there rashes, signs of local infection, swelling, abdominal distension, wounds, drains? Remember to preserve patient dignity and comfort at all times.

ⓘ Top tip

Remember to document your findings in the medical notes, and have these countersigned by your educator. Ensure that you communicate your findings and concerns to an appropriate member of the team – use SBAR to frame your handover.

17.3 Falls

Falls are a common and serious health issue in the UK, with those aged 65 years or older being at greatest risk of falling. Falls are defined as events which result in the individual unintentionally coming to rest on the ground (or lower level), but which do not have a precipitating intrinsic event such as stroke or pulmonary embolus. The consequences of falling include physical harm (including fractures), pain, loss of confidence, loss of independence and death. Of those patients who fall, 50% will fall again within 12 months.

There are many risk factors that contribute to falls – these may include: previous falls; impairments in balance/mobility/flexibility; impaired vision; effects of polypharmacy; environmental factors; confusion/agitation; certain conditions (for example Parkinson's disease, post-surgery, dementia, etc.); and frailty.

As a physiotherapy student, your role is likely to include working with the multidisciplinary team to identify risk, implement prevention strategies, conduct environmental assessments and offer appropriate exercise rehabilitation. If your placement involves working with older adults (ward or community based) you should ensure that you have completed revision on multifactorial risk assessment.

In-hospital falls are the most frequently reported safety incident, but research suggests that certain precautions may reduce these by 20–30%. If you are mobilising a patient you should consider the following:

- Baseline mobility (consider walking aids; do you need the assistance of another person?)
- Orthostatic BP
- Vision and hearing (consider spectacles and hearing aids)
- Confusion
- Toileting and continence needs
- Environment (consider footwear, clutter-free space).

What should I do if a patient falls whilst in my care?

- If a patient begins to fall whilst you are nearby, do not attempt to catch them. If it is safe for you to do so (and you have been trained) you can lower them to the floor in order to protect their head.
- Stay with the patient and call for help.
- Check their vital signs (ABCDE assessment) and assess for injuries.
- Once help has arrived, assess how to safely move the patient from the floor. If they are unable to get onto their knees and stand independently, moving and handling equipment may be required.
- Inform the patient's medical team (use SBAR communication).
- Complete an incident report as soon as possible after the event – ask your educator to help you with this to ensure that you document all the relevant information.

Chartered Society of Physiotherapy (2014) *Physiotherapy works: falls – a community approach*. Available at: bit.ly/CSP-PW

Morris, R. and O'Riordan, S. (2017) Prevention of falls in hospital. *Clinical Medicine*, **17:** 360–2.

NICE (2019) *Falls – risk assessment*. Available at: bit.ly/Falls-RA

Public Health England (2018) *Falls: applying All Our Health*. Available at: bit.ly/PHE-Falls

17.4 Sepsis

Sepsis is a life-threatening condition that arises when the body's response to an infection injures its own tissues and organs. Sepsis is caused by an infection, for example respiratory, intra-abdominal, renal, skin, joint or blood-borne. Sepsis may be complicated by septic shock when profound circulatory, cellular and metabolic abnormalities occur. Sepsis and septic shock are major global causes of morbidity and mortality.

A global initiative, the Surviving Sepsis Campaign, has established the aim of reducing mortality by 25% in 5 years, and improving awareness, diagnosis and treatment of sepsis. The Surviving Sepsis Campaign has highlighted the importance of speed in identifying and treating patients with sepsis in order to improve outcomes.

How do I identify a patient with sepsis?

Identifying a patient with sepsis can be difficult for students and trained clinicians alike – the symptoms of sepsis are very similar to many other conditions. Measuring and monitoring the patient's vital signs gives important clues – you should always report any abnormalities to a trained member of staff. Use of the National Early Warning Score (NEWS2 – see inside back cover) may help identification.

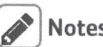 **Notes**

NICE recommends that all healthcare professionals think 'could this be sepsis?' if a person presents with signs or symptoms that indicate possible infection. The UK Sepsis Trust suggests a screening tool that may help your clinical reasoning. If all conditions are met, the patient should be screened for sepsis.

Could this be sepsis?	
Patient looks sick	✓
Patient, carer or relative very worried	✓
NEWS2 (or similar track and trigger system) triggering	✓
Risk factors present (over 75 years old, recent surgery / trauma / invasive procedure, immunosuppressed, indwelling device, or skin integrity breached)	✓

A Red Flag system identifies patients at most risk of deterioration. One or more of the following requires immediate action:

- Objective change in behaviour or mental state
- Unable to stand / collapsed
- Extremely breathless, barely able to speak
- Skin that is very pale, mottled or blue
- Rash that does not fade when firmly pressed
- Not passed urine in last 18 hours
- Recent chemotherapy.

Daniels, R. and Nutbeam, T. (eds) (2017) *The Sepsis Manual*, 4th edition. UK Sepsis Trust. Available online at: bit.ly/SM-4e

NICE (2016) *Sepsis: recognition, diagnosis and early management*. Available at: www.nice.org.uk/guidance/ng51

It is important to be familiar with different types of medications that you may come in contact with on placements. Having this knowledge may help you in understanding a patient's past medical history which may subsequently influence your own assessment, diagnosis and treatment. If you are unsure, or simply wish to learn more, ask your educator, team pharmacist (if applicable), or consult the *British National Formulary* (BNF) content available online through NICE at https://bnf.nice.org.uk.

Reason for medication (commonly referred to as)	Medication group name	Examples of some common drugs in the group
Pain relief (see *Section 18.1* for further information)	Analgesics	Paracetamol, codeine, ibuprofen
Nausea	Anti-emetic	Cyclizine, ondansetron, metoclopramide
Cholesterol-reducing	Statins	Simvastatin, lovastatin
Blood thinners	Anti-platelet drugs, anticoagulants	Warfarin, heparin, rivaroxaban, aspirin
To promote passage of urine	Diuretics	Furosemide, bendroflumethiazide
Lowering BP	Antihypertensives	Amlodipine, lisinopril, atenolol

Reason for medication (commonly referred to as)	Medication group name	Examples of some common drugs in the group
Bacterial infection	Antibiotics	Amoxicillin, erythromycin, clarithromycin, cefuroxime, metronidazole
Irregular heart rate	Anti-arrhythmics	Digoxin
Angina	Nitrates	GTN (glyceryl trinitrate)
Wheezing (bronchospasm)	Bronchodilators	Salbutamol, salmeterol, ipratropium bromide
Thick sputum	Mucolytics	Carbocysteine
Constipation	Laxatives	Docusate, senna
Depression	Antidepressants	Paroxetine, citalopram, sertraline, fluoxetine

18.1 Pain medications

Physiotherapists often treat patients who may be taking a variety of analgesic medications depending on the type of pain experienced, the severity and the level of chronicity. Be aware that there are many different ways of delivering pain medication, including oral, intramuscular, intravenous and patient-controlled analgesia.

Most people are familiar with 'over the counter' painkillers such as paracetamol or ibuprofen. You may also come across other pain medications:

Amitriptyline, pregabalin, gabapentin – neuropathic pain medications that may be used to treat either chronic pain conditions or pain that is neuropathic in nature, such as radicular pain, chronic regional pain syndrome or phantom limb pain.

Codeine, dihydrocodeine – opioid medication that may be used to treat mechanical or nociceptive pain where analgesics such as paracetamol have been unsuccessful.

Morphine, fentanyl – stronger opioid medications that may be used when weaker opioids have been unsuccessful in gaining control of pain.

Notes

It is a good idea to keep a list of other medications that you encounter during placement	
Name/type of medication	Reason for medication

NICE (2019) *BNF*. Available at: https://bnf.nice.org.uk/

Pain assessment

Pain is defined by Williams and Craig (2016, p. 2420) as *"a distressing experience associated with actual or potential tissue damage with sensory, emotional, cognitive, and social components"*. It is a complex symptom that many patients describe, and may be the reason that they seek physiotherapy treatment. It is essential that you are able to assess this subjective experience as thoroughly as possible, in order to aid your clinical reasoning.

A useful mnemonic to use is **SOCRATES** – this allows you to explore the multidimensional nature of a patient's pain experience:

Site	Where is the pain felt? Is it localised or diffuse? Can the patient point to it?
Onset	Did the pain develop suddenly or gradually? Is it continuous or intermittent? Is it improving or getting worse? What was the patient doing when the pain started?
Character	What is the nature of the pain? What words does the patient use to describe the pain, e.g. aching, agonising, crushing, cramping, pounding, stabbing, stinging, burning, shooting, etc.
Radiation	Does the pain radiate, and if so in what pattern of distribution?
Associations	Are there any other symptoms associated with the pain, e.g. dizziness, paraesthesia, breathlessness?
Time course	When did the pain first start? Is it acute or chronic? Does the pain follow any particular pattern, e.g. after exercise, after meals, worse at night?

Exacerbating / relieving factors	Can the patient describe activities or conditions that aggravate or ease the pain?
Severity	Mild / moderate / severe? Graded 0 to 10 (where 0 is no pain and 10 is unbearable)? Use of visual analogue scale? Use of FACES Pain Rating Scale?

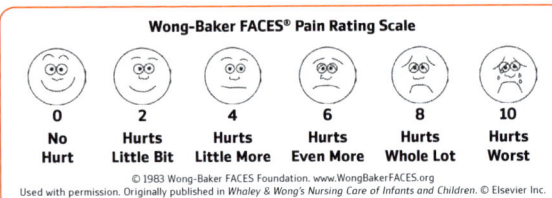

Wong-Baker FACES® Pain Rating Scale

0	2	4	6	8	10
No Hurt	Hurts Little Bit	Hurts Little More	Hurts Even More	Hurts Whole Lot	Hurts Worst

© 1983 Wong-Baker FACES Foundation. www.WongBakerFACES.org
Used with permission. Originally published in *Whaley & Wong's Nursing Care of Infants and Children.* © Elsevier Inc.

Top tip

With minor modification, the SOCRATES mnemonic can also be used to explore other symptoms such as breathlessness or fatigue.

Notes

Williams, A.C. de C. and Craig, K.D. (2016) Updating the definition of pain. *Pain,* **157**: 2420–3.

Moving on

Critical reflection describes the process of learning through and from experience – generally thinking more deeply about an experience than usually would be the case. It requires a level of self-awareness that promotes critical analysis of your own responses and assumptions in order to gain new understandings and improve your future practice. As such, critical reflection is a core pillar of your continuing professional development (CPD), and underpins clinical governance and licensing / revalidation processes. Students who practise critical reflection in healthcare education also report improved confidence, a clearer notion of professional identity and feelings of empowerment. Your clinical educators will almost certainly ask you to reflect upon your placement experiences, and you may also be asked to submit reflections as part of your course assessment.

ℹ Top tip

There will be occasions where you will participate in 'unstructured' reflections with colleagues, clinical educators or fellow students. These often happen naturally through conversation and may be thought of as a 'debrief'. As well as provoking self-awareness and learning, debriefs can be a useful way of managing emotions and stress.

In any form of reflection (structured or unstructured) remember to maintain confidentiality and preserve the anonymity of those involved.

Using a reflective framework can be a productive way to approach the reflection activity systematically and comprehensively. There are a number of frameworks commonly used by healthcare professionals, all of which aim to encourage the practitioner to think beyond simple 'description' and into levels of evaluation and analysis, such that formative conclusions can be drawn and a developmental action plan generated. A commonly used framework is Gibbs' Reflective Cycle:

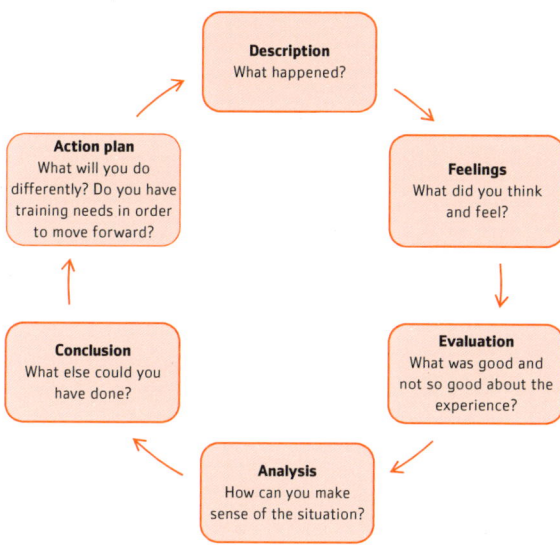

Description
What happened?

Feelings
What did you think and feel?

Evaluation
What was good and not so good about the experience?

Analysis
How can you make sense of the situation?

Conclusion
What else could you have done?

Action plan
What will you do differently? Do you have training needs in order to move forward?

Think about an event that happened recently – perhaps in the university or clinical setting, or even in a social context. Use the Gibbs' cycle to explore the experience in more detail – make sure you complete all of the steps! Think about the insights you gain from using the framework; what did you learn that might be useful in terms of your future development?

At the end of your placement, reflect on the key piece of advice you would give the next physiotherapy student placed there. For example, was there some critical pre-reading that would have made your transition into placement easier? Are there practical tips you might offer? As a cohort, get into the habit of sharing these reflective tips.

Evaluation of the placement

There is a professional expectation that you reflect upon your placement experience, and many educators will ask for verbal feedback as part of the final review. They will want to know if they provided a good learning opportunity and if you can think of any adjustments that might improve it for future students. Your placement provider and university may have formal evaluation forms that are used in order to monitor the quality of placement provision. It is important that you complete the evaluations honestly but remain professional in your comments. Both universities and placement providers value this feedback highly and use it to develop and improve placements.

Completing the evaluations can be a useful step in the process of reflecting on the placement. It may assist you to identify what types of environment you flourish in, or areas you find challenging. You can then use this knowledge to consider objectives and strategies for your next placement.

✏️ **Notes**

Gibbs, G. (1988) *Learning by Doing: a guide to teaching and learning methods.* Further Education Unit, Oxford Polytechnic.

Woolliams, M., Williams, K., Butcher, D. and Pye, J. (2009) *Be More Critical!* Oxford Brookes University. Available at: bit.ly/Brookes-2009

What happens if I make a mistake on placement?

It is really important that you inform your educator or another qualified healthcare professional as soon as possible. Depending on the nature of the incident, an incident form may need to be completed. These should not be seen as a means of attributing blame, but rather a way of identifying how future errors can be avoided. Reflecting on what happened, and why, can help you understand the situation more comprehensively and highlight relevant learning needs.

What should I do if a patient refuses to be treated by a student?

First and foremost, patients are entirely within their rights to refuse to be treated by a healthcare student. There are many reasons why a patient may refuse, and you should not ask them for justification. Sometimes it can be helpful to inform them that your work is always overseen by a qualified clinical educator, but this should be for information only and not persuasion or coercion.

How can I look after myself following an emergency or distressing situation?

Sometimes students are exposed to situations that they find extremely distressing – this could be an emergency incident (for example a cardiac arrest), a patient death, or anything else that triggers memories or causes anxiety. Do not attempt to 'battle on' – sometimes students worry that expressing their distress or anxiety may be perceived as being unprofessional. This is not the case – indeed, working whilst you are distressed is more likely to lead to mistakes, omissions and poor performance. Ask your educator, another clinician or your university tutor for a debrief session. Most universities also have counselling services that you can access if you feel that you need ongoing support.

> **What happens if I am not enjoying my placement? Or I don't get on with my educator?**

Some placements will simply be more enjoyable than others – this may be because it is an area that really interests you, or that you are working in a team that you have formed strong working relationships with. You should try to make the most of every placement, even if you feel that you are not learning as much as you could be. Take the opportunity to arrange other experiences – working with another professionals perhaps, or visiting theatre or a clinic. Interprofessional working and learning is a great way to enhance your understanding of the wider healthcare context.

If you are concerned that the placement is going badly, it is always good to raise any concerns as soon as possible. Support can be provided from a number of different sources. In the first instance you may feel able to share any concerns with your educator. You will also have a named contact from university, or your personal tutor, who you could email or phone. Many placement areas also have Practice Learning Teams whose details you will be given.

All educators will expect to see some evidence of preparatory work during your placement – this would be considered normal and not 'showing off'. They may expect to review your study notes, discuss your critical reflections or review your electronic CPD folder. Have a chat with them at the start of placement about their expectations. You may be required to complete a case study or piece of work appraising current literature during your placement – both of which are great opportunities to showcase your background work.

It is a good idea to take a folder of work with you to placement – if there are any quiet moments or gaps in your timetable you can do some background work or preparation. This is much more visible than doing work on your phone, when your educator may think you are catching up on your social media!

What should I do if I disagree with my educator regarding my mark?

There should be opportunity for you to discuss your mark with your educator so that they can justify your grades against the marking criteria. It would be fair to ask your educator what would be expected in order to achieve a higher mark.

Some universities have visiting tutors who can attend in order to help facilitate the discussion. Timely face-to-face meetings often resolve the issue. If there is no one available to visit from your university, you can contact your personal tutor for advice.

If you are still unhappy it would be worth reflecting on the situation, perhaps self-marking against the criteria. On rare occasions students may use the university grievance or appeal policy, but unless there has been an error in process it is not possible to challenge an academic or clinical mark. Remember that just working and trying hard does not always lead to high marks.

✏️ Notes

My Notes

My Notes

My Notes

My Notes

My Notes

My Notes

My Notes